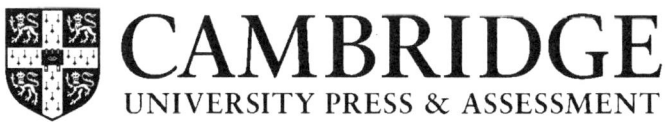

Sold To:

AMAZON.COM
HGR6
55 W. OAK RIDGE DR.
HAGERSTOWN, MD 21740-7301

ORD=Ordered Qty, SHP=Shipped Qty

QTY		TITLE	AUTHOR	ED/T
ORD	SHP			
1	1	Lean as a Healthcare Improveme	Radnor/Williams	P/P

This Document does not show any sales taxes or VAT. This is not a tax invoice.

Run No.		Lines	1
Batch/Doc	136948849	Quantity	1
Shipment No.	000288	Ship	1
Ship Via		Ship Charge	.00
Op/Doc tp		Reg Wt. lbs.	.39
Seq. No.		Cartons	1

The Chancellor, Masters, and Scholars of University of Cambridge, acting through its department Cambridge University
Cambridge University Press & Assessment, University Printing House, Shaftesbury Road, Cambridge CB2 8BS, United

Packing List

Page 1

Copy Code 1

Document No. 0083366332
Date 10/07/25
Document Type Standard Order
Customer No. 0090025593

Supply To:

AMAZON.COM
55 W. OAK RIDGE DR.
HAGERSTOWN, MD 21740-7301

ISBN	P.O. No.	PRICE	DISC %	NET VALUE
9781009326148	1WOTXLXV	23.00	35.0%	14.95

Carrier UPS GROUND COLLECT		Subtotal	14.95
Weight in Lbs. .39			
		Freight / Handling	.00
U.S. Dollar		Total	14.95

Press & Assessment. A common law Corporation by Act of Parliament in 1571.
Kingdom. Telephone 800-872-7423 Email customer_service@cambridge.org
WC 697 #RS2HR 20P0151 10/09/25 1WOTXLXV

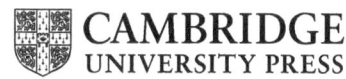
CAMBRIDGE
UNIVERSITY PRESS

Shaftesbury Road, Cambridge CB2 8EA, United Kingdom

One Liberty Plaza, 20th Floor, New York, NY 10006, USA

477 Williamstown Road, Port Melbourne, VIC 3207, Australia

314–321, 3rd Floor, Plot 3, Splendor Forum, Jasola District Centre, New Delhi – 110025, India

103 Penang Road, #05–06/07, Visioncrest Commercial, Singapore 238467

Cambridge University Press is part of Cambridge University Press & Assessment, a department of the University of Cambridge.

We share the University's mission to contribute to society through the pursuit of education, learning and research at the highest international levels of excellence.

www.cambridge.org
Information on this title: www.cambridge.org/9781009326148
DOI: 10.1017/9781009326124

© THIS Institute 2025

This publication is in copyright. Subject to statutory exception and to the provisions of relevant collective licensing agreements, with the exception of the Creative Commons version the link for which is provided below, no reproduction of any part may take place without the written permission of Cambridge University Press & Assessment.

An online version of this work is published at doi.org/10.1017/9781009326124 under a Creative Commons Open Access license CC-BY-NC-ND 4.0 which permits re-use, distribution and reproduction in any medium for non-commercial purposes providing appropriate credit to the original work is given. You may not distribute derivative works without permission. To view a copy of this license, visit https://creativecommons.org/licenses/by-nc-nd/4.0

When citing this work, please include a reference to the DOI 10.1017/9781009326124

First published 2025

A catalogue record for this publication is available from the British Library

ISBN 978-1-009-32614-8 Paperback
ISSN 2754-2912 (online)
ISSN 2754-2904 (print)

Cambridge University Press & Assessment has no responsibility for the persistence or accuracy of URLs for external or third-party internet websites referred to in this publication and does not guarantee that any content on such websites is, or will remain, accurate or appropriate.

Every effort has been made in preparing this Element to provide accurate and up-to-date information which is in accord with accepted standards and practice at the time of publication. Although case histories are drawn from actual cases, every effort has been made to disguise the identities of the individuals involved. Nevertheless, the authors, editors and publishers can make no warranties that the information contained herein is totally free from error, not least because clinical standards are constantly changing through research and regulation. The authors, editors and publishers therefore disclaim all liability for direct or consequential damages resulting from the use of material contained in this Element. Readers are strongly advised to pay careful attention to information provided by the manufacturer of any drugs or equipment that they plan to use.

For EU product safety concerns, contact us at Calle de José Abascal, 56, 1°, 28003 Madrid, Spain, or email eugpsr@cambridge.org

Cambridge Elements

Elements of Improving Quality and Safety in Healthcare
edited by
Mary Dixon-Woods,* Katrina Brown,* Sonja Marjanovic,†
Tom Ling,† Ellen Perry,* Graham Martin,* Gemma Petley,*
and Claire Dipple*
*THIS Institute (The Healthcare Improvement Studies Institute)
†RAND Europe

LEAN AS A HEALTHCARE IMPROVEMENT APPROACH

Zoe Radnor[1] and Sharon J. Williams[2]
[1] College of Business and Social Sciences, Aston University
[2] School of Health and Social Care, Faculty of Medicine, Health and Life Science, Swansea University

THIS.Institute — The Healthcare Improvement Studies Institute

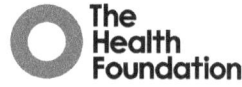

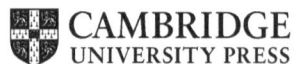

Lean as a Healthcare Improvement Approach

Elements of Improving Quality and Safety in Healthcare

DOI: 10.1017/9781009326124
First published online: September 2025

Zoe Radnor[1] and Sharon J. Williams[2]
[1]College of Business and Social Sciences, Aston University
[2]School of Health and Social Care, Faculty of Medicine, Health and Life Science, Swansea University

Author for correspondence: Zoe Radnor, z.radnor@aston.ac.uk

Abstract: Lean is one of the most widely used improvement approaches in healthcare. With origins in manufacturing, it focuses on improving efficiency, eliminating waste, and streamlining processes. This Element provides an overview of the evidence for the use of Lean in healthcare, summarises the supporting tools and techniques, and emphasises the importance of developing an organisational culture committed to continuous improvement. The authors offer two case studies of attempts to implement Lean at scale, noting that, despite its popularity, implementation is not straightforward. Challenges include terminology that isn't always easy to grasp, perceived dissonances between the manufacturing origins of Lean based on repetitive, standardised, automated production and the human-centred world of healthcare, and problems with fidelity. The authors make the case that there is a lack of a robust evidence base for Lean and call for well-designed studies to advance the implementation of Lean and associated process improvement techniques in healthcare. This title is also available as open access on Cambridge Core.

Keywords: Lean, process improvement, Six Sigma, Lean Six Sigma, implementation

© THIS Institute 2025

ISBNs: 9781009326148 (PB), 9781009326124 (OC)
ISSNs: 2754-2912 (online), 2754-2904 (print)

Contents

1 Introduction   1
2 Lean in Action   5
3 Implementing Lean   10
4 Critiques of Lean in Healthcare   12
5 Conclusions   14
6 Further Reading   15

  Contributors   16
  References   18

1 Introduction

This Element focuses on Lean, one of the most widely used improvement approaches.[1] The term 'Lean' was first coined in 1988 by Krafcik[2] to explain the success of the Toyota Production System in simultaneously achieving high levels of productivity and quality in Japanese car production. Womack et al.'s 1990 book *The Machine That Changed the World*[3] is often seen as having popularised Lean. Womack and Jones' text *Lean Thinking*,[4] published in 1996, was particularly influential in emphasising that a key feature of Lean is a focus on eliminating *waste* – defined as any part of a process that adds time, effort or cost, but no direct value. *Lean Thinking* proposed five key principles (Box 1), based on the underlying assumption that organisations are made up of processes, and that using these principles in a stepwise and sequential way can add value, reduce waste, and continuously improve in an ever-repeating process.[5]

A large volume of academic and practitioner writing has emerged since the 1990s, but – despite its widespread use – no single consensus on a definition of Lean has emerged.[6,7] Generally speaking, however, Lean comprises a 'philosophy' of ideas and principles and a set of tools, techniques, and practices aimed at reconfiguring organisational processes to reduce waste and enhance productivity. It involves the systematic and rigorous application of a range of specialist improvement tools, techniques, and frameworks,[8,9,10] coupled with a culture of continuous improvement.[11] Accordingly, one useful definition is:

> *Lean as a management practice based on the philosophy of continuously improving processes by either increasing customer value or reducing non-value-adding activities (*muda*), process variation (*mura*), and poor work conditions (*muri*).*[5]

Blended approaches that combine Lean with other improvement approaches have also appeared. Among the most popular of these is Lean Six Sigma:[1,12,13] a hybrid of Lean and Six Sigma. Six Sigma is a business process improvement methodology, characterised by a set of statistical and management tools (e.g. cause-and-effect diagrams, Pareto analysis, process maps, and data collection). A prominent feature of Six Sigma is its use of 'projects', typically using a methodology known as DMAIC (Define, Measure, Analyse, Improve, and Control). It has been argued that combining Lean and Six Sigma offers a powerful means of improving productivity and efficiency by reducing waste and variation.[14]

1.1 Lean in Healthcare

Despite its origins in manufacturing, Lean can be used in any organisation where processes can be mapped, goals measured, and resources managed.[7]

> **BOX 1: WOMACK AND JONES' FIVE KEY PRINCIPLES OF LEAN**
>
> 1. Specify the value desired by the customer.
> 2. Identify the value stream for each product/service providing that value and challenge all non-value-adding steps.
> 3. Make the product flow continuously. Standardise processes around best practice, allowing them to run more smoothly, freeing up time for creativity and innovation.
> 4. Introduce 'pull' between all steps where continuous flow is impossible. Focus on the demand from the customer and trigger process steps backwards through the value chain.
> 5. Strive towards perfection so that non-value-adding activity will be removed from the value chain, meaning that the number of steps, amount of time and information needed to serve the customer continually reduces.

Interest in the potential of Lean in healthcare is long-standing and enduring.[15] The Lean philosophy of putting the customer first, its focus on quality and safety, and its commitment to employees is part of the appeal,[16] but so too is the potential for the approach to support management of capacity and demand,[17,18] as well as waste and flow.[6] Toussaint and Gerard's *On the Mend*,[19] published in 2010, set out something of a manifesto for Lean in healthcare, based on principles including focusing on the patient, designing care around the patient, identifying value for the patient, removing waste, improving the flow for patients, providing information and materials, and reducing time to treatment.

Like Lean in other sectors, Lean in healthcare focuses on reducing waste, typically by studying a process and eliminating, rationalising, or reducing the steps deemed to be wasteful. While Lean is customarily described as being concerned with seven types of waste, healthcare adds an eighth – the waste of human potential when frontline health workers are not heard, engaged, or supported to improve (Table 1). However, a focus on waste alone is overly restrictive, given that *muda* (waste) is only one of three interrelated concepts in Lean. *Mura* relates to 'unevenness' and argues for stable demand that results in less variation and more efficient and standardised processes, while *muri* relates to 'excessive strain', and argues for good working conditions.[5]

Lean activities can usefully be divided into three categories according to their purpose: assessment, improvement, and monitoring (Table 2). The tools and techniques used to support Lean in other industries can all, in principle, be used

Table 1 The 'seven wastes' found in manufacturing and corresponding examples in healthcare

Original seven wastes[20]	Examples of healthcare wastes[21]
Transportation	Unnecessary transportation and moving of patients and equipment
Inventory	Over-stocking of clinical and non-clinical supplies; tests awaiting processing or distribution
Motion	Looking for missing patient information; sharing medical equipment
Waiting (delay)	Staff waiting for equipment; patients waiting to be seen; patients waiting for results; patients waiting for take-home medicines
Over-production	Requesting unnecessary diagnostic tests
Over-processing	Producing excessive documentation or duplication of documentation
Defects	Prescription errors; incorrect information; incorrect diagnosis
The eighth waste in healthcare: the under-utilisation of human potential	Staff not working to the full scope of their role, grade, or registration, meaning that their improvement insights and potential are wasted

Adapted from Ohno[20] and Guimarães and Carvalho[21]

in healthcare;[22] Costa and Filho's 2016 review identified around 24 Lean tools and methods in use in healthcare settings.[23]

Importantly, Lean is not just about tools and techniques but also about the organisational culture and leadership.[5] For activities to be effective, the organisational culture needs to be informed by a philosophy of continuous improvement, involving all employees at all levels. *Kaizen*, a Japanese term meaning 'continuous improvement', involves both specific activities and a cultural commitment to improvement. Focused leadership appears to be particularly important for Lean,[25] and is characterised by behaviour patterns and routines that focus not just on doing the work or delivering the service but also improving the work.[26,27] Proudlove and Furnival[28] suggest that improvement *kata* – an approach that breaks down a vision into a set of achievable target conditions – can be used to develop Lean management behaviour and make scientific

Table 2 Types of Lean activities classified by purpose

Type of Lean activity	Example
Assessment Reviewing and mapping existing organisational processes in terms of their waste, flow, or capacity to add value.	**A3** A 10-step method using a single sheet of A3 paper to characterise the problem, background, current condition, goal, root cause, target condition, counter-measures, implementation plan, test, and follow-up.
Improvement Supporting and improving processes through redesign, using problem-solving and other methods.	**5S** Seeking to organise the work area by: • Sorting: eliminating anything not needed • Straightening: organising the remaining items • Shining: cleaning and inspecting the work area • Standardising: writing standards • Sustaining: regularly applying the standards
Monitoring Enabling measurement of any improvements.	**Statistical process control** Using specific methods to characterise 'common cause' variation – inherent in the process – and 'special cause' variation – which operates outside of that process (see the Element on statistical process control).[24]

problem-solving habitual to form the foundations for solid and ongoing healthcare improvement.

While continuous improvement involves an ongoing commitment, not a single one-off intervention, Lean often involves specific improvement efforts. They might typically start with a '*kaizen* blitz' or 'rapid improvement' event involving a small team of frontline professionals. Perhaps held over 3–5 days, such events might be the first step in an effort to record and evaluate a current process, develop and design a new process, and review results. The team will seek first to understand value – particularly as defined by patients. Next, the team will seek to characterise the processes as they currently operate. Often, this will involve what is called *gemba* ('real place') to observe what happens in practice, including any inefficiencies, frustrations, duplications, gaps, and so on. This analysis is used to populate a value stream map – the set of steps or actions that takes place in a process or patient journey, including the length of time it takes to complete the process (lead time) and the time taken to complete each step (process time). Value stream mapping is best understood as a diagnostic technique that describes the present status of a process, with the output known as a current state value stream map (CSVSM).

After this, a 'flow' state is visualised, where the improvement team seeks to identify how all the steps in the process might follow each other seamlessly. This will typically involve generating ideas for how the various steps might be streamlined or improved (including elimination of unnecessary steps and redesign or reimagining of other steps), which are then synthesised and depicted on a future state value stream map (FSVSM). This idealised future state is then used as the basis of the next step: an improvement plan. Specifying responsibilities for implementation, and perhaps involving improvement coaches, the plan should recognise that change is not easy, that resistance and challenges are likely, and that leadership support will be necessary. The implementation phase will involve multiple tests of change that can be used to optimise flow and progress towards the future state. Finally, pursuing perfection requires that all colleagues seek to improve every day, supported by an organisational commitment to continuous improvement.

2 Lean in Action

Lean has been widely used in healthcare, particularly in acute care (hospitals), to address issues such as waiting times, workflow,[29,30] and operational efficiencies.[31,32,33] Examples of Lean Six Sigma are also reported in the literature,[31] motivated by concerns such as improving patient safety, increasing operational efficiency, and reducing financial costs.[34]

In this section, we offer two case studies of attempts to implement Lean at scale in the National Health Service (NHS) in the UK: the Productive Ward Programme and the Virginia Mason Production System.

2.1 Case Study 1: Productive Ward – National Improvement Programme

The NHS Institute for Innovation and Improvement's 'Productive Series' is a prominent example of an effort to introduce Lean into a healthcare system.

The Productive Ward: Releasing Time to Care programme was developed in 2005 and piloted with four test sites in 2006 and then with a further ten learning partners during 2007–08. It focused on streamlining ward processes, improving the ward environment, and thereby increasing time for face-to-face patient contact.[35] In May 2008, the UK government provided a £50 million investment to support the rollout of the Productive Ward initiative more widely in England.[18] Built on principles of Lean thinking,[36] the package consisted of guidance for leaders at project, ward, and executive levels, together with 11 self-directed learning modules:

- Three foundation modules: Knowing how we are doing, Well-organised ward, and Patient status at a glance.
- Eight process modules: including areas such as improving shift handovers, mealtimes, and medicine rounds.
- One toolkit.

The Productive Ward 'package' became an international programme, and similar programmes were developed for other specialisms, including Productive Operating Theatre, Productive Mental Health Ward, and Productive General Practice.[37]

Studies reporting on the programme suggested benefits for staff and patients. Reported improvements related to time spent directly on patient care, nurse handover time, and time taken for medicine rounds,[38] as well as reductions in the amount of time staff spent doing tasks unrelated to patient care, and culture change in using specialist knowledge to improve quality of services.[39] However, the study designs used to evaluate Productive Ward were mostly weak and lacking in suitable comparators or control, making it difficult to draw conclusions about the effectiveness of the programme.

Studies examining implementation of Productive Ward found that it was often challenging. For example, Robert et al.'s[40] multi-methods study looking at the ten-year impact in six hospitals identified that fidelity was often problematic, and that the time-limited funding (two years) was insufficient to support hospital-wide implementation. Resource constraints and a managerial preference for standardisation were seen to influence a move away from the original goal of empowering ward staff to take ownership of the programme towards taking shortcuts on the implementation. Even within hospitals, there was considerable variation between wards in how the programme was implemented. Nonetheless, some legacies of the Productive Ward programme were identified, such as the display of metrics (e.g. number of falls or infections on a ward), management of ward supplies and equipment, and practices like protected mealtimes.[40]

> **BOX 2: CONTEXTUAL CHARACTERISTICS OF PRODUCTIVE WARD IMPLEMENTATION**
>
> 1. Engaging in a robust communication strategy to support the implementation and spread of the programme.
> 2. Enabling and empowering facilitators and ward leaders to implement and spread the programme.
> 3. Making appropriate training and support available to those involved in the programme.
> 4. Using good project planning and project management to support the timely implementation of the programme.
> 5. Clear role for all leaders to clarify responsibilities and accountability.
> 6. Giving continued executive and management engagement and support.
> 7. Providing financial and human resource commitments to support the implementation and spread of the programme.
>
> Adapted from White et al. 2014[41]

White et al.'s review of 53 articles[41] identified 7 contextual characteristics (Box 2) that influence implementation, several of them previously identified to some extent in the change and implementation literature.[42,43]

One feature that emerged strongly from the scholarship on the Productive Ward was the extent of commitment and leadership required from senior management. Bloodworth,[44] for example, highlighted the need for the progress of the Productive Ward programme to be monitored via a steering group chaired by the chief executive.

The Productive Ward programme was introduced nearly two decades ago. Although some elements have been sustained in the NHS, there is little to suggest that the programme has fully achieved its goals.

2.2 Case Study 2: Virginia Mason Production System

In 2002, the Virginia Mason Medical Center in the United States began developing the Virginia Mason Production System. Modelled on the Toyota Production System and principles of Lean thinking, it aimed to secure the highest level of safety, improved care delivery, and elimination of waste.[16] In 2008, in response to growing demand from healthcare organisations worldwide to understand and apply Lean methods, the Virginia Mason Institute – a non-profit organisation specialising in healthcare transformation – was founded. Since then, many organisations have attempted to emulate the Virginia Mason Production System, though often with mixed results.[45–48]

In 2015, a five-year partnership was set up between NHS Improvement and the Virginia Mason Institute to support five NHS trusts in England.[49] Each trust was asked to work with the Virginia Mason Institute and NHS Improvement (a then-extant arm's-length body) to develop localised versions of the Virginia Mason Production System and to build a sustainable culture of continuous improvement capability across each organisation.

The programme featured training/education at various levels, including a 'train the trainer' programme. At the end of the third year, all trusts reported that they were able to coach and train their own staff in improvement methods.[50]

The programme also featured support for using Lean methods, including *kaizen*-style rapid improvement events.[48,51] Involving a small, dedicated team working over 3–5 days to analyse and improve a narrowly defined quality issue or process, each participating NHS trust was able to decide which care pathways they wanted to improve and how to go about it – including what measures to use and at what level (e.g. organisation, clinic). Table 3 gives examples of the value streams selected by the participating trusts and any improvements they reported making.

An independent mixed-method evaluation of the partnership,[51] was undertaken in 2018–2021, part of which covered some of the COVID-19 pandemic period.[51] Although all sites within the Virginia Mason Institute programme were found to have made some improvements, particularly in process lead times,[51,52] the evaluation report provides a mixed picture in terms of the level of progress and success across sites.[52] All five trusts achieved significant overall reductions in process lead times, though the reductions were variable. Organisation-wide improvement was not straightforward, with some improvements restricted to specific care pathways or services. While three of the trusts were reported to have achieved wide-scale improvements that improved their financial position, quality of care, and staff morale, two were placed in special measures – meaning that their performance was deemed inadequate.[51]

The evaluation identified that a strong culture of peer learning and knowledge sharing was a key enabler of organisation-wide improvement. The more successful organisations invested time and resource in encouraging and empowering staff to share their ideas and knowledge with others, as well as being willing to learn from each other, and this appears to have made a difference. As might be anticipated, visible and sustained commitment from leaders was needed to gain organisation-wide traction and support. Those who viewed the programme largely as a technical exercise involving a few experts working alongside frontline staff were less likely to fully embed the programme within the organisation. Organisations that were able to view the programme as core to the organisation's identity and strategic vision had a greater likelihood of the

Table 3 Value streams and impact

Trust	Value stream	Improvement/impact
Shrewsbury and Telford Hospital NHS Trust	Recruitment	• 68 days' reduction in the time taken between a vacancy being identified to a new member of staff starting. • 20 days' reduction in the number of days taken to get a job applicant's reference. • 13 per cent reduction in non-clinical agency staff.
University Hospitals Coventry and Warwickshire NHS Trust	Surgery/ anaesthesia	• 63 per cent reduction in the time taken to get patients ready for anaesthetic.
Barking, Havering and Redbridge University Hospitals NHS Trust	Cancer	• Reduction in time taken to prepare suspected cancer biopsy samples for analysis from 22 hours to 5 hours.
Leeds Teaching Hospitals NHS Trust	Urology surgery	• Reduction in time taken to discharge some patients following specialist urology surgery from 39 hours to 24 hours.
Surrey and Sussex Healthcare NHS Trust	Outpatients	• Reduction in time taken to process medical records in preparing clinic lists for the day from 41 minutes to nine minutes. • Reduction in number of steps walked by patient having blood test from 212 to 18.

Burgess, Currie, Crump, and Dawson[51]

programme being embedded and having a greater impact.[52] Trusts that had the highest Care Quality Commission (CQC) ratings were found to have greater levels of social connectedness between staff than those with the lowest ratings, indicating that priority needs to be given to allowing staff to come together on a regular basis to share ideas and learning in an open and respectful way.[52] High-quality measurement was one of the most demanding parts of the programme (see the Element on measurement for improvement).[53] It was reported to have improved during the programme as trusts got better at being able to select appropriate metrics for each level,[52] but clearly requires attention in any improvement programme.

3 Implementing Lean

Despite the enthusiasm for Lean, it is clear that its implementation in healthcare is not straightforward.[54–63] One challenge for Lean is that its terminology, including Japanese terms for concepts such as *muda* (waste) and *gemba* (real place), is not always easy to grasp. A deeper problem, perhaps, is the potential for dissonance between the world of manufacturing, based on highly repetitive, automated production of repeatable items, and the human-centred world of healthcare.[64] Also challenging is the perceived link between Lean and efforts to reduce resources and staff,[65] leading to some reluctance to use the term Lean. There has also been a corresponding emergence of other terms, such as Model of Improvement and Virginia Mason Production System, that often share much in common with Lean but are not called Lean.

A second challenge is that implementing Lean may need long-term organisational policies and strategic planning; a switch from a hierarchical culture to an improvement culture that supports workforce stability, team leadership and decentralised decision-making; and recognition of the socio-technical nature of healthcare work.[61,64] The available evidence suggests that Lean in healthcare needs to integrate technical elements (such as tools and workplace layout) and social elements (such as teamwork, organisational culture, employee learning, and participation).[61] Sustainability also requires Lean to be viewed as more than a set of projects, but instead as an ongoing way of approaching work and thinking about systems.[5,66,67]

In practice, there is a tendency to give significant attention to Lean tools and techniques[61,68] but reducing Lean to a toolbox risks reducing recognition of the need for the cultural change and leadership behaviours required to deliver improvement.[69] Many would argue that the tools and techniques have dominated the implementation discussion over the important aspect of behavioural and culture change.[70–73] Joosten et al.,[67] for example, report that when the emphasis is process-oriented, little attention may be given to context and the human side of improvement. Even when the emphasis is on tools and techniques, fidelity of implementation is often problematic.[73]

A further challenge lies in the level of senior leadership and management commitment required to support the strategic alignment of organisations with Lean practices and philosophies, as illustrated by both the Productive Ward and

Virginia Mason case studies. It is noted by van Elp et al.[25] that the role of management is a key ingredient for improvement in healthcare, but, while the concept of Lean leadership is discussed in the literature,[74] understanding of how different leadership styles impact on Lean and improvement more generally is limited, especially in relation to leadership behaviours.[75] A multi-case, multi-methods study in the Netherlands found that a hybrid leadership approach is likely to be required in order for Lean implementation to be successful. This approach combines leadership behaviours that are transactional (based on extrinsic rewards and give-and-take relationships) and transformational (inspiring others to buy in to a strategic vision and go beyond self-interest) and appeared to promote the improvement capability of teams.[18]

Further, as the two case studies demonstrate, Lean and other improvement approaches rely heavily on staff involvement and commitment.[76,77] Disengagement of staff has been reported as the biggest reason for Lean failure,[78] but monitoring and enhancing of Lean team experience and satisfaction are often overlooked.[70] McCann et al.'s three-year study[78] of the introduction of Lean in a large UK hospital found initial enthusiasm for the approach, especially at ward level, but scepticism and reservations about the approach later appeared. Practical barriers included heavy workloads, insufficient resources, and not being able to take staff away from their clinical duties to attend meetings and training. Many of the improvement interventions were superficial, both in relation to their impact and their connection to Lean, and there was sporadic use of improvement tools that were labelled as Lean but might not have been. Limited progress 'led to Lean appearing weak, pliable and superficial'.[79]

A further challenge for Lean implementation is the tendency for efforts to focus on specific departments (e.g. accident and emergency) rather than the entire healthcare organisation.[76,80] Small, localised improvements may help organisations to maintain momentum, but there is a risk of sub-optimising other parts of the wider health and social care system.[81] Even within single organisations, failing to take a systems improvement approach may mean that an improvement in one area can simply move an issue (e.g. waiting times) elsewhere.[82]

Linked to these kinds of challenges, Lean and other improvement approaches may be adopted in healthcare in a piecemeal fashion before being abandoned in favour of the latest initiative without allowing time to embed.[83,84] The 'readiness' of the organisation not only to implement but also to maintain their adopted approach is crucial.[85,86] Some scholars advocate that understanding the local context is crucial when implementing Lean in healthcare.[54,87] Yet important attributes of context are often poorly defined, and current knowledge of the role of contextual factors in implementing new practices and methods such as Lean is limited.[49,88,89]

4 Critiques of Lean in Healthcare

Lean is widely discussed and deployed in health services globally and enjoys widespread engagement, belief, support, and commitment. However, it is also clear that it faces a number of challenges. Some of these relate to the lack of a robust evidence base for Lean. By 2009, Brandão de Souza's review[90] had identified over 90 academic articles from ten different countries, which classified studies into three areas:

- Manufacturing-type cases – improvements to manufacturing or process environments, such as radiology or pharmacy.
- Support services cases – improvements in areas such as IT, human resources, and finance.
- Patient flow cases – improvements to length of stay and waiting list initiatives.

This review identified reports of improvements in areas such as waiting times and reduction of errors and costs,[91] as well as intangible benefits such as increased employee motivation.[5] Other studies since then have documented the continued popularity of Lean in healthcare,[92] in areas as diverse as surgery, emergency departments, mental health, and pharmacy. Some reviews continue to report improvements arising from the use of Lean,[43] including reductions in errors or defects and variability, better physical layout, and the optimisation of resource allocation and inventory.[62,93] Reduction in time (e.g. length of stay and release of test results) is the most reported benefit.[94,95,96]

However, much of the research on Lean in health settings is characterised by poor quality study designs. There appears to be an overreliance on single site, pathways, or service case studies. Robust and well-structured evaluations are rare, tending to be missing altogether or done too early. Moraros et al.'s review[57] of 22 articles found that none used high-quality experimental study designs such as randomised control trials or quasi-experimental study designs (e.g. prospective longitudinal cohorts). Only four reported on health outcomes, and just one of these found a statistically significant impact of implementing Lean. A total of fifteen studies focusing on process outcomes covered areas such as waiting times, patient flow, and workplace engagement, but only two found a statistically significant positive effect of Lean. None of the 22 studies reported on the financial costs.

The lack of longitudinal studies has further limited insight.[97,98] Lean interventions are often reviewed over a period of 1–2 years,[99] potentially offering little understanding of the impact and sustainability of Lean over the longer term.[84,97,100,101] As the Productive Ward case study illustrates, many organisations report short-term gains when implementing Lean, but more widespread and sustained improvements may be elusive. Similarly, a review of Lean Six Sigma studies showed that only 20 per cent of studies reported on the long-term (1–3 years) effects of the improvement. To help evidence the sustainability of these studies, a longitudinal post-intervention period is required.[31] There is a clear need to use methods other than single-case studies, such as pre- and post-interventions and ethnographic studies.[62]

The ability to show the strategic and whole-systems impact of Lean and Lean Six Sigma[31] has been especially lacking, linked to the tendency for implementation to be pragmatic, patchy, and fragmented.[66] A Lean healthcare system should operate as a cohesive and well-connected system rather than as a collection of independent facilities.[102] However, Burgess and Radnor's[22] evaluation of Lean in English NHS trusts found that implementation tended to be isolated rather than system-wide, leading to a disjointed approach. The problems stem from how healthcare organisations are functionally organised, often characterised by fragmentation,[103] but also how implementation tends to be approached.

A perhaps fundamental challenge regarding the evidence base is that, although understanding the value of the 'customer' (patient) is central to the principles of Lean in healthcare, there is limited research to show how the value or the voice of the customer/patient[104] is captured and used within Lean and associated approaches,[73] and evidence of direct benefit for patients has been slow to appear. Similarly, how Lean integrates with the person-centred and co-production agenda is also unclear. Although both synergies and divergences have been noted between Lean Six Sigma and person-centred care,[105] further research is required to identify where and how Lean and associated techniques can enhance patient care and transform person-centred cultures.

More well-designed, applied studies using the principles of evidence-based medicine are needed to assure the quality and credibility of the evidence base for Lean. Bateman reminds us that interdisciplinary research can strengthen most fields of enquiry, especially in improving and managing healthcare quality, but also emphasises the need for an appreciation of the idiosyncrasies of the sector, including professional dynamics.[106] Learning from other disciplines outside healthcare will help us to continue to progress understanding of healthcare improvement. Theory-based evaluations are likely to be helpful, as illustrated by an evaluation of a six-year single Lean case study that used Programme

Theory to help understand and capture cultural, individual, and team influences on the Lean interventions.[107] Well-designed studies should also clearly identify what adaptations are needed to accommodate the nuances and intricacies of our healthcare systems. These studies would benefit from the discipline of operations management but also other theoretical lenses (such as psychology, sociology, and design science) to understand the complexity and interdependence of healthcare settings. Longitudinal studies, especially post-intervention, are needed to evidence the sustainability of improvements achieved and to identify when outcomes start to wane. Approaches such as simulation[100] may help in developing systems-level evaluation. Benefits realisation frameworks based on quality, time, and cost[102] would help to create the evidence base and give confidence in the healthcare improvements achieved through utilising a Lean-based approach, as many healthcare professionals make a diagnosis through data.

Finally, much of the Lean and the Lean Six Sigma literature focuses on hospitals and acute healthcare. More studies are needed to evidence how Lean and Lean Six Sigma are implemented within community and primary care settings. Further research into Lean and associated techniques is also needed for integrated networks that include social care.

5 Conclusions

In this Element, we have both acknowledged the popularity of Lean in healthcare and reported on its mixed results using case studies and the broader literature. It is clear that a strong evidence base of well-designed studies is imperative to advance the implementation of Lean and associated process improvement techniques in healthcare. Future research should use study designs that are regarded as powerful from the perspective of evidence-based medicine (e.g. including well-designed observational, experimental, and quasi-experimental designs with a longitudinal emphasis). However, research should also draw more widely on other disciplines (such as psychology, sociology, medicine), as well as industrial and operational management, given the need to investigate the sociotechnical elements required for the implementation of Lean and to develop the necessary conceptual model for further testing.[62] This should also extend to research into how Lean and Lean Six Sigma can be used with new emerging trends and technologies (such as artificial intelligence, automation, and robotics) as they are introduced and embedded within our healthcare systems.[34] Similarly, recognising how Lean can be integrated with other established improvement models, approaches, and frameworks would be useful.

Learning from the negative impacts of implementing Lean also needs to be analysed and reported to advance our understanding of Lean in healthcare.[62]

6 Further Reading

Graban[102] – provides a practical insight to the implementation of Lean in a hospital setting.

Bicheno[108] – explains how various Lean tools can be used within service organisations.

Radnor[8] – compares key approaches, such as Lean and Six Sigma.

Radnor et al.[109] – provide case chapters on various aspects of improving healthcare operations, including a Lean case study.

Contributors

Both authors have contributed equally. Both authors have approved the final version.

Conflicts of Interest

None.

Acknowledgements

We thank the THIS Institute editorial team and the peer reviewers for their insightful comments and recommendations to improve the Element. A list of peer reviewers is published at www.cambridge.org/IQ-peer-reviewers.

Funding

This Element was funded by THIS Institute (The Healthcare Improvement Studies Institute, www.thisinstitute.cam.ac.uk). THIS Institute is strengthening the evidence base for improving the quality and safety of healthcare. THIS Institute is supported by a grant to the University of Cambridge from the Health Foundation – an independent charity committed to bringing about better health and healthcare for people in the UK.

About the Authors

Zoe Radnor is Pro Vice-Chancellor at Aston University. Zoe has led research projects for government and healthcare organisations, evaluating the use of Lean. Zoe is a Principal Fellow of Higher Education (PFHEA), a Fellow of the Academy of Social Sciences (FAcSS) and British Academy of Management (FBAM). She sits on Boards including Liverpool Institute of Performing Arts (LIPA).

Sharon J. Williams is Professor of Healthcare Operations Management at Swansea University and visiting Professor with the College of Business and Social Sciences at Aston University. Her background is in service operations and supply chain management, and her interdisciplinary research aims to improve the quality of health and social care services by drawing on approaches used in other sectors.

Creative Commons License

The online version of this work is published under a Creative Commons licence called CC-BY-NC-ND 4.0 (https://creativecommons.org/licenses/by-nc-nd/4.0). It means that you're free to reuse this work. In fact, we encourage it. We just ask that you acknowledge THIS Institute as the creator, you don't distribute a modified version without our permission, and you don't sell it or use it for any activity that generates revenue without our permission. Ultimately, we want our work to have impact. So if you've got a use in mind but you're not sure it's allowed, just ask us at enquiries@thisinstitute.cam.ac.uk.

The printed version is subject to statutory exceptions and to the provisions of relevant licensing agreements, so you will need written permission from Cambridge University Press to reproduce any part of it.

All versions of this work may contain content reproduced under licence from third parties. You must obtain permission to reproduce this content from these third parties directly.

References

1. Henrique D, Filho M. A systematic literature review of empirical research in Lean and Six Sigma in healthcare. *Total Qual Manag Bus Excell* 2020; 31(3–4): 429–49. https://doi.org/10.1080/14783363.2018.1429259.
2. Krafcik J. Triumph of the Lean production system. *Sloan Manage Rev* 1988; 30(1): 41–52.
3. Womack J, Jones D, Roos D. *The Machine that Changed the World*. New York: Macmillan; 1990.
4. Womack J, Jones D. *Lean Thinking: Banish Waste and Create Wealth in Your Corporation*. New York: Simon Schuster; 1996.
5. Radnor ZJ, Holweg M, Waring J. Lean in healthcare: The unfilled promise? *Soc Sci Med* 2012; 74(3): 364–71. https://doi.org/10.1016/j.socscimed.2011.02.011.
6. Shah R, Ward P. Defining and developing measures of Lean production. *J Oper Manag* 2007; 25(4): 785–805. https://doi.org/10.1016/j.jom.2007.01.019.
7. Samuel D, Found P, Williams S. How did the publication of the book *The Machine that Changed the World* change management thinking? Exploring 25 years of Lean literature. *Int J Oper Prod Manag* 2015; 35(10): 1386–407. https://doi.org/10.1108/IJOPM-12-2013-0555.
8. Radnor ZJ. *Review of Business Process Improvement Methodologies in Public Services*. London: Advanced Institute of Management Research; 2010. www.researchgate.net/publication/266868980_Review_of_Business_Process_Improvement_Methodologies_in_Public_Services (accessed 14 June 2021).
9. Ogden G, Moncy B. *Lean Healthcare: Creating a Lean-Thinking Culture*. Waukesha, WI: GE Healthcare; 2009. www.canhealth.com/WhitePapers/GE_Lean_White_Paper.pdf (accessed 14 June 2023).
10. Hines P, Found P, Harrison R. *Staying Lean: Thriving, Not Just Surviving*. Cardiff: Lean Enterprise Research Centre, Cardiff University; 2008. https://orca.cardiff.ac.uk/id/eprint/52764/1/stayinglean.pdf (accessed 14 June 2021).
11. Langley GL, Nolan KM, Nolan TW, Norman CL, Provost LP. *The Improvement Guide: A Practical Approach to Enhancing Organizational Performance, 2nd ed*. San Francisco, CA: Jossey Bass; 2009.
12. Vaishnavi V, Suresh M. Modelling of readiness factors for the implementation of Lean Six Sigma in healthcare organizations. *Int J Lean Six Sigma* 2020; 11(4): 597–633. https://doi.org/10.1108/IJLSS-12-2017-0146.

13. Kuiper A, Lee RH, van Ham VJJ, Does RJMM. A reconsideration of Lean Six Sigma in healthcare after the COVID-19 crisis. *Int J Lean Six Sigma* 2022; 13(1): 101–17. https://doi.org/10.1108/IJLSS-01-2021-0013.
14. George ML. *Lean Six Sigma: Combining Six Sigma Quality with Lean Production Speed.* New York: McGraw-Hill; 2002.
15. Santos ACSG, Reis AC, Souza CG, Santos IL, Ferreira LAF. The first evidence about conceptual vs analytical lean healthcare research studies. *J Health Organ Manag* 2020; 34(7): 789–806. https://doi.org/10.1108/JHOM-01-2020-0021.
16. Bohmer R, Ferlins E. *Virginia Mason Medical Center.* Boston, MA: Harvard Business School 2005; 3: 1–28. https://hbsp.harvard.edu/product/606044-PDF-ENG (accessed 14 June 2021).
17. Walley P. Does the public sector need a more demand-driven approach to capacity management? *Prod Plan Control* 2013; 24(10–11): 877–90. https://doi.org/10.1080/09537287.2012.666886.
18. Walley P, Jennison-Phillips A. A study of non-urgent demand to identify opportunities for demand reduction. *J Pol Pract* 2020; 14(2): 542–54. https://doi.org/10.1093/police/pay034.
19. Toussaint J, Gerard R. *On the Mend.* Cambridge, MA: Lean Enterprise Institute; 2010.
20. Ohno T. *Toyota Production Systems: Beyond Large Scale Production.* Cambridge, MA: Productivity Press; 1988.
21. Guimarães C, Carvalho J. Strategic outsourcing: A Lean tool of healthcare supply chain management. *SOIJ* 2013; 6(2): 138–66. https://doi.org/10.1108/SO-11-2011-0035.
22. Burgess N, Radnor Z. Evaluating Lean in healthcare. *Int J Health Care Qual Assur* 2013; 26(3): 220–35. https://doi.org/10.1108/09526861311311418.
23. Costa LBM, Filho MG. Lean healthcare: Review, classification and analysis of literature. *Prod Plan Control* 2016; 27(10): 823–36. https://doi.org/10.1080/09537287.2016.1143131.
24. Mohammed MA. Statistical process control. In Dixon-Woods M, Brown K, Marjanovic S et al., editors. *Elements of Improving Quality and Safety in Healthcare.* Cambridge: Cambridge University Press; 2024. https://doi.org/10.1017/9781009326834.
25. Van Elp B, Roemeling O, Aij KH. Lean leadership: Towards continuous improvement capability in healthcare. *Health Serv Manage Res* 2022; 35(1): 7–15. https://doi.org/10.1177/09514848211001688.
26. Rother M. *Toyota Kata: Managing People for Improvement, Adaptiveness and Superior Results.* New York: McGraw-Hill; 2010.

27. Rother M. *Toyota Kata Practice Guide*. New York: McGraw-Hill; 2018.
28. Proudlove N, Furnival J. Toyota Kata: A missing link in quality improvement in healthcare? In *University of Manchester: Proceedings of the 27th European Operations Management Association Conference*. EurOMA27. 2020; 1818–27. www.research.manchester.ac.uk/portal/files/173909338/EurOMA_full_1.5.pdf (accessed 14 June 2021).
29. Hynes JP, Murray AS, Murra OM et al. Use of Lean Six Sigma methodology shows reduction of inpatient waiting time for peripherally inserted central catheter placement. *Clin Radiol* 2019; 74(9): 718–43. https://doi.org/10.1016/j.crad.2019.04.022.
30. Godley M, Jenkins JB. Decreasing wait times and increasing patient satisfaction. *J Nurs Care Qual* 2019; 34(1): 61–65. https://doi.org/10.1097/NCQ.0000000000000332.
31. Samanta AK, Gurumurthy A. Implementing Lean Six Sigma in health care: A review of case studies. *Int J of Lean Six Sigma* 2023; 14(1): 158–89. https://doi.org/10.1108/IJLSS-08-2021-0133.
32. Devi BI, Shukla DP, Bhat DI et al. Neurotrauma care delivery in a limited resource setting – Lessons learned from referral and patient flow in a tertiary care center. *World Neurosurg* 2019; 123: e588–e596. https://doi.org/10.1016/j.wneu.2018.11.227.
33. Molla M, Warren DS, Stewart SL et al. A Lean Six Sigma quality improvement project improves timeliness of discharge from the hospital. *Jt Comm J Qual Patient Saf* 2018; 44(7): 401–12. https://doi.org/10.1016/j.jcjq.2018.02.006.
34. McDermott O, Antony J, Bhat S et al. Lean Six Sigma in healthcare: A systematic literature review on motivations and benefits. *Processes* 2022; 10(10): 1910. https://doi.org/10.3390/pr10101910.
35. Robert G, Morrow E, Maben J, Griffiths P, Callard L. The adoption, local implementation and assimilation into routine nursing practice of a national quality improvement programme: The Productive Ward in England. *J Clin Nurs* 2011; 20: 1196–207. https://doi.org/10.1111/j.1365-2702.2010.03480.x.
36. Bevan H. How can we build skills to transform the healthcare system? *J Nurs Res* 2010; 15(2): 139–48. https://doi.org/10.1177/1744987109357812.
37. NHS Institute for Innovation and Improvement (NHSII) (2011). The Productive Series. www.england.nhs.uk/improvement-hub/wp-content/uploads/sites/44/2017/11/The-Productive-Series-generic-flyer.pdf.
38. Wilson G. Implementation of releasing time to care – The Productive Ward. *J Nurs Manag* 2009; 17: 647–54. https://doi.org/10.1111/j.1365-2834.2009.01026.x.

39. Bloodworth K. The Productive Ward and the Productive Operating Theatre. *J Perioper Pract* 2011; 21(3): 97–103. https://doi.org/10.1177/175045891102100303.
40. Robert G, Sarre S, Maben J, Griffiths P, Chable R. Exploring the sustainability of quality improvement interventions in healthcare organisations: A multiple methods study of the 10-year impact of the 'Productive Ward: Releasing Time to Care' programme in English acute hospitals. *BMJ Qual Saf* 2020; 29: 31–40. http://dx.doi.org/10.1136/bmjqs-2019-009457.
41. White M, Wells J, Butterworth T. The Productive Ward: Releasing Time to Care™ – What we can learn from the literature for implementation. *J Nurs Manage* 2013; 22: 914–23. https://doi.org/10.1111/jonm.12069.
42. Ferlie EB, Shortell SM. Improving the quality of health care in the United Kingdom and the United States: A framework for change. *Milbank Q* 2001; 79: 281–315. https://doi.org/10.1111/1468-0009.00206.
43. Kotter J. Leading change: Why transformation efforts fail. *Harv Bus Rev* 2007; 85(1): 96–103. https://hbr.org/2007/01/leading-change-why-transformation-efforts-fail.
44. Bloodworth K. Productive Ward 1: Implementing the initiative across a large university teaching hospital. *Nurs Times* 2009; 105: 24. www.nursingtimes.net/news/hospital/productive-ward-1-implementing-the-initiative-across-a-large-university-teaching-hospital-22-06-2009 (accessed 14 June 2021).
45. Pham H, Ginsburg P, McKenzie K, Milstein A. Redesigning care delivery in response to a high-performance network: The Virginia Mason Medical Center. *Health Aff* 2007; 26: 532–44. https://doi.org/10.1377/hlthaff.26.4.w532.
46. Hunter D, Erskine J, Hicks C et al. A mixed-methods evaluation of transformational change in NHS North East. *National Institute for Health Research* 2014; 2(47): 1–218. https://doi.org/10.3310/hsdr02470.
47. Erskine J, Hunter D, Hicks C et al. New development: First steps towards an evaluation of the North East Transformation System. *Public Money Manag* 2009; 29: 273–6. https://doi.org/10.1080/09540960903205857.
48. Hunter D, Erskine J, Small A et al. Doing transformational change in the English NHS in the context of 'big bang' redisorganisation: Findings from the North East transformation system. *J Health Organ Manag* 2015; 29: 10–24. https://doi.org/10.1108/JHOM-01-2014-0019.
49. Burgess N, Richmond J. *Evaluation of the NHS Partnership with Virginia Mason Institute, End of First Year Report – Executive Summary*. Warwick: Warwick Business School; 2019.

50. Jacobson G. Which works better, Kaizen events or daily Kaizen? KaiNexus blog; 2015. https://blog.kainexus.com/improvement-disciplines/kaizen/kaizen-events/kaizen-events-vs-daily-kaizen (accessed 14 June 2023).
51. Burgess N, Currie G, Crump B, Dawson A. *Leading Change across a Healthcare System: How to Build Improvement Capability and Foster a Culture of Continuous Improvement, Report of the Evaluation of the NHS-VMI Partnership*. Warwick: Warwick Business School; 2022. https://warwick.ac.uk/fac/soc/wbs/research/vmi-nhs/reports/report_-_leading_change_across_a_healthcare_system_22.09.2022.pdf.
52. Jones, B. *Building an Organisational Culture of Continuous Improvement: Learning from the Evaluation of the NHS Partnership with Virginia Mason Institute*. Health Foundation; 2022. www.health.org.uk/reports-and-analysis/briefings/building-an-organisational-culture-of-continuous-improvement.
53. Toulany A, Shojania K. Measurement for improvement. In Dixon-Woods M, Brown K, Marjanovic S et al., editors. *Elements of Improving Quality and Safety in Healthcare*. Cambridge: Cambridge University Press; 2025. https://doi.org/10.1017/9781009326063.
54. Parkhi SS. Lean management practices in healthcare sector: A literature review. *Benchmarking Int J* 2019; 26(4): 1275–89. https://doi.org/10.1108/BIJ-06-2018-0166.
55. Poksinska B. The current state of Lean implementation in health care: Literature review. *Qual Manag Health Care* 2010; 19(4): 319–29. https://doi.org/10.1097/QMH.0b013e3181fa07bb.
56. LaGanga L. Lean service operations: Reflections and new directions for capacity expansion in outpatient clinics. *J Oper Manag* 2011; 29(5): 422–33. https://doi.org/10.1016/j.jom.2010.12.005.
57. Moraros J, Lemstra M, Nwankwo C. Lean interventions in healthcare: Do they actually work? A systematic literature review. *Int J Qual Health Care* 2016; 28(2): 150–65. https://doi.org/10.1093/intqhc/mzv123.
58. D'Andreamatteo A, Ianni L, Lega F, Sargiacomoa M. Lean in healthcare: A comprehensive review. *Health Policy* 2015; 119: 1197–1209. https://doi.org/10.1016/j.healthpol.2015.02.002.
59. Hallam C, Contreras C. Lean healthcare: Scale, scope and sustainability. *Int J Health Care Qual Assur* 2018; 31(7): 684–96. https://doi.org/10.1108/IJHCQA-02-2017-0023.
60. Salentijn W, Beijer S, Antony J. Exploring the dark side of Lean: A systematic review of the lean factors that influence social outcomes. *TQM J* 2021; 33(6): 1469–83. https://doi.org/10.1108/TQM-09-2020-0218.

61. Marsilio M, Pisarra M. Lean management in health care: A review of reviews of socio-technical components for effective impact. *J Health Organ Manag* 2021; 35(4): 475–91. https://doi.org/10.1108/JHOM-06-2020-0241.
62. Santos ACSG, Reis AC, Souza CG et al. Measuring the current state-of-the-art in Lean healthcare literature from the lenses of bibliometric indicators. *Benchmarking* 2023; 30(9): 3508–33. https://doi.org/10.1108/BIJ-10-2021-0580.
63. Deblois S, Lepanto L. Lean and Six Sigma in acute care: A systematic review of reviews. *Int J Health Care Qual Assur* 2016; 29(2): 192–208. https://doi.org/10.1108/IJHCQA-05-2014-0058.
64. Spear S. Fixing healthcare from the Inside: Teaching residents to heal broken delivery processes as they heal sick patients. *Acad Med* 2006; 81(10): 144–9. https://doi.org/10.1097/00001888-200610001-00034.
65. Adler PS, Goldoftas B, Levine DI. Flexibility versus efficiency? A case study of model changeovers in the Toyota production system. *Organ Sci* 1999; 10: 43–68. https://doi.org/10.1287/orsc.10.1.43.
66. Young T, McClean S. A critical look at Lean thinking in healthcare. *Qual Saf Health Care* 2008; 17: 382–6. https://doi.org/10.1136/qshc.2006.020131.
67. Joosten T, Bongers I, Janssen R. Application of Lean thinking to healthcare: Issues and observations. *Int J Qual Health Care* 2009; 21(5): 341–7. https://doi.org/10.1093/intqhc/mzp036.
68. Reed J, Card A. The problem with plan-do-study-act cycles. *BMJ Qual Saf* 2015; 2: 147–52. http://dx.doi.org/10.1136/bmjqs-2015-005076.
69. Camuffo A, Fabrizio G. Modeling management behaviors in Lean production environments. *Int J Oper Prod Manage* 2018; 38(2): 403–23. https://doi.org/10.1108/IJOPM-12-2015-0760.
70. Stone K. Four decades of lean: A systematic literature review. *Int J Lean Six Sigma* 2012; 3(2): 112–32. https://doi.org/10.1108/20401461211243702.
71. Camuffo A, Gerli F. Modeling management behaviors in Lean production environments. *Int J Oper Prod Manage* 2018; 38(2): 403–23. https://doi.org/10.1108/IJOPM-12-2015-0760.
72. Dixon-Woods M, Martin G. Does quality improvement improve quality? *Future Hosp J* 2017; 3(3): 191–4. https://doi.org/10.7861/futurehosp.3-3-191.
73. Radnor Z, Osborne S. Lean: A failed theory for public services? *Public Manag Rev* 2013; 15(2): 265–87. https://doi.org/10.1080/14719037.2012.748820.
74. Ward A, Liker JK, Cristiano JJ, Sobeck DK. The second Toyota paradox: How delaying decisions can make better cars faster. *Sloan Manag Rev*

1995; 36: 43–61. https://sloanreview.mit.edu/article/the-second-toyota-paradox-how-delaying-decisions-can-make-better-cars-faster/ (accessed 15 April 2022).
75. Poksinska B. The current state of Lean implementation in health care: Literature review. *Qual Manag Health Care* 2010; 19: 319–29. https://doi.org/10.1097/QMH.0b013e3181fa07bb.
76. Tlapa D, Zepeda-Lugo C, Tortorella G et al. Effects of Lean healthcare on patient flow: A systematic review. *Value in Health* 2020; 23(2): 260–73. https://doi.org/10.1016/j.jval.2019.11.002
77. Hines P, Taylor D, Walsh A. The Lean journey: Have we got it wrong? *Total Qual Manag Bus Excell* 2020; 31(3–4): 389–406. https://doi.org/10.1080/14783363.2018.1429258.
78. Albanese C, Aaby D, Platchek T. *Advanced Lean in Healthcare*. North Charleston, SC: Create Space Independent Publishing Platform; 2014.
79. McCann L, Hassard J, Granter E, Hyde P. Casting the lean spell: The promotion, dilution and erosion of lean management in the NHS. *Hum Relat* 2015; 68(10): 1557–77. https://doi.org/10.1177/0018726714561697.
80. Sommer AC, Blumenthal EZ. Implementation of Lean and Six Sigma principles in ophthalmology for improving quality of care and patient flow. *Surv Ophthalmol* 2019; 64(5): 720–8. https://doi.org/10.1016/j.survophthal.2019.03.007.
81. Ronen B, Pliskin J, Pass, S. *The Hospital and Clinic Improvement Handbook: Using Lean and the Theory of Constraints for Better Healthcare Delivery*. Oxford: Oxford University Press; 2018.
82. Leite H, Williams S, Radnor Z, Bateman N. Emergent barriers to the Lean healthcare journey: Baronies, tribalism and scepticism. *Prod Plan Control* 2022; 35(2): 115–32. https://doi.org/10.1080/09537287.2022.2054386.
83. Proudlove N, Moxham C, Boaden R. Lessons for Lean in healthcare from using Six Sigma in the NHS. *Public Money Manag* 2008; 28(1): 27–34.
84. Jabbal J. Embedding a culture of quality improvement. London: The Kings Fund; 2017. www.kingsfund.org.uk/publications/embedding-culture-quality-improvement.
85. Leite H, Bateman N, Radnor Z. Beyond the ostensible: An exploration of barriers to lean implementation and sustainability in healthcare. *Prod Plan Control* 2019; 31(1): 1–18. https://doi.org/10.1080/09537287.2019.1623426.
86. Williams SJ, Radnor ZJ. Moving from service to sustainable services: A healthcare case study. *Int J Product Perform Manag* 2022; 71(4): 1126–48. https://doi.org/10.1108/IJPPM-12-2019-0583.

87. Chassin MR. Improving the quality of health care: What's taking so long? *Health Aff* 2013; 32(10): 1761–5. https://doi.org/10.1377/hlthaff.2013.0809.
88. Rangachari P. Innovation implementation in the context of hospital QI: Lessons learned and strategies for success. *Innov Entrep Health* 2018; 5: 1–14. https://doi.org/10.2147/IEH.S151040.
89. Reponen E, Rundall T, Shortell S et al. Benchmarking outcomes on multiple contextual levels in lean healthcare: A systematic review, development of a conceptual framework, and a research agenda. *BMC Health Serv Res* 2021; 21: 161. https://doi.org/10.1186/s12913-021-06160-6.
90. Brandão De Souza L. Trends and approaches in Lean healthcare. *Leadersh Health Serv* 2009; 22(2): 121–39. https://doi.org/10.1108/17511870910953788.
91. Silvester K, Lendon R, Bevan H, Steyn R, Walley P. Reducing waiting times in the NHS: Is lack of capacity the problem? *Clin Manag* 2004; 12(3): 105–11.
92. Jiang W, Sousa PSA, Moreira MA, Amaro GM. Lean direction in literature: A bibliometric approach. *Prod Manuf Res* 2021; 9(1): 241–63. https://doi.org/10.1080/21693277.2021.1978008.
93. Abdallah AB, Alkhaldi RZ. Lean bundles in health care: A scoping review. *J Health Organ Manage* 2019; 33(4): 488–510. https://doi.org/10.1108/JHOM-09-2018-0263.
94. Mousavi Isfahani H, Tourani S, Seyedin H. Lean management approach in hospitals: A systematic review. *Int J Lean Six Sigma* 2019; 10(1): 161–88. https://doi.org/10.1108/IJLSS-05-2017-0051.
95. Vest JR, Gamm LD. A critical review of the research literature on Six Sigma, Lean and StuderGroup's hardwiring excellence in the United States: The need to demonstrate and communicate the effectiveness of transformation strategies in healthcare. *Implement Sci* 2009; 1(4): 35. https://doi.org/10.1186/1748-5908-4-35.
96. Woodnutt S. Is Lean sustainable in today's NHS hospitals? A systematic literature review using the meta-narrative and integrative methods. *Int J Qual Health Care* 2018; 30(8): 578–86. https://doi.org/10.1093/intqhc/mzy070.
97. Mazzocato P, Thor J, Backman U et al. Complexity complicates lean: Lessons from seven emergency services. *J Health Organ Manag* 2014; 28(2): 266–88. https://doi.org/10.1108/JHOM-03-2013-0060.
98. Stentoft J, Freytag P. Improvement culture in the public mental healthcare sector: Evaluation of implementation efforts. *Prod Plan Control* 2020; 31(7): 540–56. https://doi.org/10.1080/09537287.2019.1657978.

99. Fillingham D. Can Lean save lives? *Leadersh Health Serv* 2007; 20(4): 231–41. https://doi.org/10.1108/17511870710829346.
100. Hallam C, Contreras C. Lean healthcare: Scale, scope and sustainability. *Int J Health Care Qual Assur* 2018; 31(7): 684–96. https://doi.org/10.1108/IJHCQA-02-2017-0023.
101. Roemeling O, Land M, Ahaus K. Does Lean cure variability in health care? *Int J Oper Prod Manage* 2017; 37(9): 1229–45. https://doi.org/10.1108/IJOPM-07-2015-0452.
102. Graban M. *Lean Hospitals – Improving Quality, Patient Safety, and Employee Engagement, 3rd ed*. London: Taylor & Francis Group; 2016.
103. Bateman N, Lethbridge S. Managing operations and teams visually. In Bell E, Warren S, Schroeder JE, editors. *The Routledge Companion to Visual Organization*. Oxford: Routledge; 2014. https://doi.org/10.4324/9780203725610.
104. Found P, Harrison R. Understanding the Lean voice of the customer. *Int. J. Lean Six Sigma* 2012; 3(3): 251–67. https://doi.org/10.1108/20401461211282736.
105. Teeling SP, Dewing J, Baldie D. A discussion of the synergy and divergence between Lean Six Sigma and person-centred improvement sciences. *Int J Res Nurs* 2020; 11: 10–23. https://doi.org/10.3844/ijrnsp.2020.10.23.
106. Bateman N. Effective use of interdisciplinary approaches in healthcare quality: Drawing on operations and visual management. *BMJ Qual Saf* 2024; 33(4): 216–19. https://doi.org/10.1136/bmjqs-2023-016947.
107. Lindsay CF, Aitken J. Using programme theory to evaluate Lean interventions in healthcare. *Prod Plan Control* 2022; 35(8): 824–41. https://doi.org/10.1080/09537287.2022.2139778.
108. Bicheno J. *The Lean Toolbox for Service Systems*. Buckingham: Picsie Books; 2008.
109. Radnor Z, Bateman N, Esain A et al. *Public Service Operations Management*. Abingdon: Routledge; 2015. https://doi.org/10.4324/9781315747972.

Cambridge Elements

Improving Quality and Safety in Healthcare

Editors-in-Chief
Mary Dixon-Woods
THIS Institute (The Healthcare Improvement Studies Institute)

Mary is Director of THIS Institute and is the Health Foundation Professor of Healthcare Improvement Studies in the Department of Public Health and Primary Care at the University of Cambridge. Mary leads a programme of research focused on healthcare improvement, healthcare ethics, and methodological innovation in studying healthcare.

Graham Martin
THIS Institute (The Healthcare Improvement Studies Institute)

Graham is Director of Research at THIS Institute, leading applied research programmes and contributing to the institute's strategy and development. His research interests are in the organisation and delivery of healthcare, and particularly the role of professionals, managers, and patients and the public in efforts at organisational change.

Executive Editor
Katrina Brown
THIS Institute (The Healthcare Improvement Studies Institute)

Katrina was Communications Manager at THIS Institute, providing editorial expertise to maximise the impact of THIS Institute's research findings. She managed the project to produce the series until 2023.

Editorial Team
Sonja Marjanovic
RAND Europe

Sonja is Director of RAND Europe's healthcare innovation, industry, and policy research. Her work provides decision-makers with evidence and insights to support innovation and improvement in healthcare systems, and to support the translation of innovation into societal benefits for healthcare services and population health.

Tom Ling
RAND Europe

Tom is Head of Evaluation at RAND Europe and President of the European Evaluation Society, leading evaluations and applied research focused on the key challenges facing health services. His current health portfolio includes evaluations of the innovation landscape, quality improvement, communities of practice, patient flow, and service transformation.

Ellen Perry
THIS Institute (The Healthcare Improvement Studies Institute)
Ellen supported the production of the series during 2020–21.

Gemma Petley
THIS Institute (The Healthcare Improvement Studies Institute)
Gemma is Senior Communications and Editorial Manager at THIS Institute, responsible for overseeing the production and maximising the impact of the series.

Claire Dipple
THIS Institute (The Healthcare Improvement Studies Institute)
Claire is Editorial Project Manager at THIS Institute, responsible for editing and project managing the series.

About the Series
The past decade has seen enormous growth in both activity and research on improvement in healthcare. This series offers a comprehensive and authoritative set of overviews of the different improvement approaches available, exploring the thinking behind them, examining evidence for each approach, and identifying areas of debate.

Cambridge Elements

Improving Quality and Safety in Healthcare

Elements in the Series

Governance and Leadership
Naomi J. Fulop and Angus I. G. Ramsay

Health Economics
Andrew Street and Nils Gutacker

Approaches to Spread, Scale-Up, and Sustainability
Chrysanthi Papoutsi, Trisha Greenhalgh, and Sonja Marjanovic

Statistical Process Control
Mohammed Amin Mohammed

Values and Ethics
Alan Cribb, Vikki Entwistle, and Polly Mitchell

Design Creativity
Gyuchan Thomas Jun, Sue Hignett and P. John Clarkson

Supply Chain Management
Sharon J. Williams

Measurement for Improvement
Alene Toulany and Kaveh G. Shojania

Learning Health Systems
Thomas Foley and Leora I. Horwitz

Clinical Microsystems and Team Coaching
Steve Harrison, Rachael Finn and Marjorie M. Godfrey

Audit, Feedback, and Behaviour Change
Noah Ivers and Robbie Foy

Lean as a Healthcare Improvement Approach
Zoe Radnor and Sharon J. Williams

A full series listing is available at: www.cambridge.org/IQ

For EU product safety concerns, contact us at Calle de José Abascal, 56–1°, 28003 Madrid, Spain or eugpsr@cambridge.org.

www.ingramcontent.com/pod-product-compliance
Lightning Source LLC
Chambersburg PA
CBHW070811091025
33787CB00023B/293